CW00721897

Magic of Eucalyptus Oil

Uses   *Hints*   *Recipes*

Cherie de Haas and Peter Abbott

INFORMATION
AUSTRALIA

Published by
Information Australia
A.C.N. 006 042 173
75 Flinders Lane
Melbourne Vic. 3000
Telephone: (03) 9654 2800
Fax: (03) 9650 5261
Internet: www.infoaust.com
Email: mail@infoaust.com

The National Library of Australia
Cataloguing-in-Publication entry:

De Haas, Cherie.
    Magic of eucalyptus oil : uses, hints, recipes.

    ISBN 1 86350 308 0

    1. Eucalyptus oil. 2. Eucalyptus oil - Therapeutic use.
    I. Abbott, Peter S. II. Title

615.32376

Page Layout & Design: Ben Graham

Printed in Australia by McPherson's Printing Group

A tribute to

Joseph Bosisto

1827 - 1898

The Australian pioneer who, in 1852, was the first
to produce eucalyptus oil commercially and who
spent the next 45 years fostering its use worldwide.

Foreword - My love of eucalyptus oil

Working as a natural therapist for over 25 years has allowed me the greatest of all honours: to be working with, and hopefully helping, many people.

I have seen many changes over the years, and the huge return to independent health. At times the market place seems inundated with claims on goods that really are not what they claim to be.

One product that has been beside me the whole time is Bosisto's Eucalyptus Oil. I grew up with it, as did my children, and it certainly has survived the test of time.

The uses I have discovered I can do with it are absolutely endless. From warding off creepy crawlies, making lotions and potions, to cleaning the clinic, it is something I use more than once a day - everyday.

One of my outside interests is treating race horses. Many years ago a patient's horse became ill and he found conventional treatments were not quite doing what he had hoped. For a time he combined both complementary treatments with conventional treatment, and was impressed with the results. That was the beginning of visiting many stables and properties, and always with my eucalyptus oil, herbal compounds, and creams.

Animals, as well as humans, respond to nature's remedies - sometimes it may take a little longer, but the results can be astounding.

At no time do I recommend you self-treat every ailment. Make sure you seek professional advice at all times, or, if what you are doing is not working, make sure you check it out.

I sincerely hope that you enjoy making these formulas, and get the results that you are looking for. Be patient – the rewards can be well worth it.

Yours in good health, always, Cherie.

Contents

About the authors

Cherie de Haas

Cherie has been in natural therapies for over 25 years and has seen many great changes, particularly where people are turning to things 'natural'.

Cherie was the first naturopath in Australia to have a segment on prime-time television, Healthy Wealthy & Wise, where she remained for seven years. She presented on Channel 10 FCTV with Julia Zaetta and Penny Cook on how to make your own skin care and home remedies.

Cherie started on radio in 1980, and is currently on 3AK each week. She has contributed articles to many magazines, and is contributing to Family Circle

(Murdoch magazines) and contributing to Hair, Body and Beauty magazine.

Cherie has a book on Natural Skin Care, now in its second edition, which, when first released in 1984, went to the International Market.

She lectures all over the world and in Australia, to corporations such as QANTAS, and the business sector.

Cherie de Haas is the mother of two children who are both involved in the family business. Her daughter, Monique runs the clinic; her son Ren, the skin care company.

Peter Abbott

Peter is Executive Chairman of his company Felton Grimwade & Bickford Pty Ltd, which is the owner of Bosisto's 'Parrot' Brand Eucalyptus Oil. Peter has been involved in eucalyptus oil production, processing, formulating and marketing since 1974.

The history of Felton Grimwade & Bickford can be traced back to 1867 when pharmacists Frederick Grimwade and Alfred Felton formed the wholesale druggist business Felton Grimwade & Co.

Joseph Bosisto was a friend of the partners and he engaged them to distribute his eucalyptus oil. In 1882, Bosisto, Felton and Grimwade formed a partnership to expand production of eucalyptus oil to meet the growing world demand.

When Bosisto died in 1898, Felton Grimwade became owners of Bosisto's 'Parrot' Brand Eucalyptus Oil.

When Alfred Felton died in 1904 leaving no dependants, his estate of nearly £400,000 was divided between charities (especially destitute women and children) and funds to purchase works of art for the National Gallery of Victoria. The Felton Bequest has formed the basis of major acquisitions of works of art in the National Gallery of Victoria and amounts to many millions of dollars so far.

The Grimwade family were also great philanthropists and in 1933 they purchased Captain Cook's cottage in Great Ayton, Yorkshire, and shipped it to Melbourne. It was re-erected in the Fitzroy Gardens and is still a major tourist attraction today.

Since Peter acquired Felton Grimwade & Bickford the company has successfully revitalised its eucalyptus operations and launched a number of innovative products which have been well received by trade outlets and consumers. The company is one of the two largest producers of eucalyptus oil in Australia. It is the only company to incorporate its eucalyptus oil into a wide range of its own products.

Peter is a Fellow of the Australian Institute of Company Directors and a Certified Practising Accountant. He has considerable experience in management and marketing in Australia and overseas. He was formerly a public company director and senior executive.

Peter's wife Alison is Felton Grimwade & Bickford's Director of Consumer Relations, son Colin is Director Marketing Services and daughter Tegan, who is at university, works as a part-time research assistant.

Introduction

Bosisto's 'Parrot' Brand Eucalyptus Oil is a natural oil distilled from the leaves of a unique Australian eucalyptus tree known as 'blue mallee'. It is an amazing natural product with multiple personal and household uses. It has been an Australian household favourite for almost 150 years.

Bosisto's 'Parrot' Brand Eucalyptus Oil is truly a 'magical' product. It can relieve the symptoms of colds and flu – sore throat, hacking cough, stuffy nose and clears nasal passages making it easier to breathe freely. It soothes and penetrates the skin to ease arthritic and muscular aches and pains.

Bosisto's 'Parrot' Brand Eucalyptus Oil is a strong antiseptic and germicidal disinfectant. It is also an excellent deodoriser and sanitiser. It is a powerful cleaner solvent and penetrating oil. It is wonderful for getting out stubborn stains and grease marks from clothes and carpets.

Eucalyptus oil is marvellous in the wash for cleaning and freshening and it has the fresh, clean fragrance of the Australian bush.

Bosisto's 'Parrot' Brand Eucalyptus Oil is an important and colourful part of Australia's history. It was the first truly Australian product and Australia's first distinctive export.

Expanding markets and several exciting potential new uses suggest its future will be even brighter than its past.

Eucalyptus Trees

The characteristic fresh fragrance of Australian eucalypt forests comes from the leaves giving off some of their eucalyptus oil.

Eucalypts form about three quarters of the tree flora of Australia.

There are over 500 species of eucalypts and all have eucalyptus oil in their leaves. The quantity and type of eucalyptus oil varies from species to species.

All eucalyptus oils are not the same. The oil from each species has different constituents and chemical composition. However, eucalyptus oil from the same species is usually remarkably constant in its constituents and chemical composition.

Only about 20 species of eucalypts have been found to have enough oil of economic value to be produced commercially. At the present time less than 10 species account for the entire world production.

As a general rule, good oil-producing species are of little use as timber, whereas those utilised for timber contain very little oil.

Eucalypts are widely distributed over the Australian continent. They range from the dwarfed and stunted forms called 'mallees' to the tall trees which grow in coastal and mountainous regions.

Eucalypts are typically Australian, although a few species have been found in neighbouring countries. The extensive plantations in North and South America, Europe, Africa, China and India were planted with Australian seeds.

The eucalypt belongs to the *Myrtaceae* family. The genus was named *Eucalyptus* by the Frenchman L'Heretier in 1788. The word came from the Greek *eu* 'well' and *kalypto* 'I cover' and refers to the cap that covers the flower buds until the buds mature and force the cap open.

Ever wondered why eucalypts are often called 'gums'? William Dampier in 1688 noted that trees in north-west Australia exuded a kind of gum. Aborigines used this gum to fasten barbs to the ends of spears and fishing sticks. The exudation from the bark which looks like a 'gum' is actually a tannin-like substance known as 'kino'. Governor Arthur Philip is credited with being the first to call the eucalypt a 'gum tree' in 1788. Since then, most Australians have called eucalypts 'gum trees'. There is nothing more Australian than a 'gum tree'!

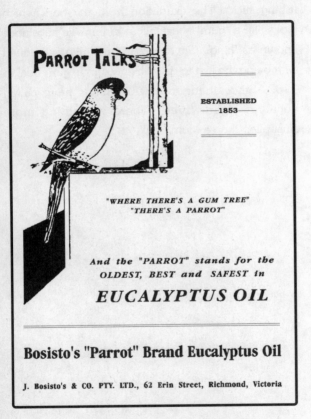

Advertisement from 'The Gum Tree', 1925.

The History Of Eucalyptus Oil

The eucalyptus oil story began in 1788 with the arrival of the First Fleet and Surgeon-General John White. Within a few weeks of arriving, White recorded in his diary the olfactory oil in the eucalyptus. Governor Arthur Philip sent a sample to Sir Joseph Banks in England.

In 1790, Surgeon-General White distilled a quart of oil from a eucalypt he called 'Sydney Peppermint' because its oil closely resembled that of peppermint, *mentha piperita*, which grows in England. He sent the quart of oil to Thomas Wilson in England for further experimentation.

When the oil was tested in England, it was reported to be *'much more efficacious in removing all cholicky complaints than that of the oil obtained from the well known English peppermint, being less pungent and more aromatic'*.

Following this discovery, other people extracted eucalyptus oil, including the pioneer Dr Robert Officer, a ship's surgeon who set up a eucalyptus still in Hobart in the 1830's. However, none exploited the opportunity commercially.

Commercial development of eucalyptus oil

Joseph Bosisto, a Victorian pharmacist, encouraged by Baron Ferdinand von Meuller, the famous government botanist of Victoria, began investigation of the commercial production of eucalyptus oil in 1852.

Joseph Bosisto was a Yorkshireman who had qualified as a pharmacist in Leeds and London. He arrived in Adelaide in 1848 at the age of 21. In 1851, he moved to Victoria in search of gold but after a few months at Castlemaine without success, he opened a pharmacy in Richmond where he built a laboratory to investigate the medicinal and chemical properties of Australian plants.

As a result of Bosisto's collaboration with von Mueller, the eucalyptus oil industry was born. Bosisto commenced operations in a small, rudely constructed still at Dandenong Creek, Victoria, using the leaves of a form of *Eucalyptus radiata* (then known as *E. amygdalina*) which grew profusely in the district. Bosisto soon built other distilleries at nearby Emerald, Menzies Creek and Macclesfield.

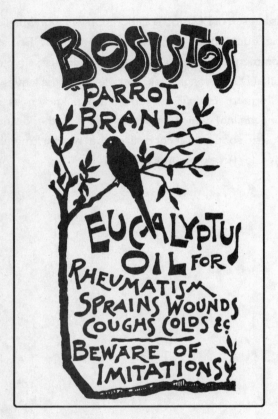

Bosisto's Parrot Brand Eucalyptus Oil
famous for almost 150 years.

Joseph Bosisto C.B.E.

Joseph Bosisto was undoubtedly among the great Australian pioneers. As well as being the first commercial producer of eucalyptus oil, Bosisto was an active promoter of the first Pharmaceutical Society in 1857. Bosisto was the first vice-president of the society and gave the inaugural address. Bosisto was also the first president of the Pharmacy Board in 1877. He became an honorary member of the Medical Society of Victoria in 1878.

Bosisto was Mayor of Richmond 1864-1866. He was also a magistrate and was chairman of the Bench for six years. He was elected to Parliament where he became a very active member from 1874 to 1889 and again in 1892. He was heavily involved with the Great Exhibitions of 1880 and 1888.

Bosisto and Felton Grimwade

Sales of Bosisto's Eucalyptus Oil were to a restricted local market until overseas interest grew sufficiently for Bosisto to begin exports to England in 1865. Messrs Alfred Felton and Frederick Grimwade saw the possibilities of the trade and their firm, Felton Grimwade & Co, became the distributors of Bosisto's Oil of Eucalyptus which then was the only distinctively Australian substance in the British Pharmacopoeia.

To develop the new industry, Felton, Grimwade, Bosisto and others formed a new firm, the Eucalyptus Mallee Company, and bought Antwerp Station – a property on the Wimmera River, near Dimboola Victoria.

In 1885, the Antwerp company was merged with Bosisto's original business and a firm called J. Bosisto and Co. was formed. The new company was to be solely a manufacturer, with Felton Grimwade and Co undertaking distribution and all the necessary bookkeeping and marketing.

Development of international markets

Sales of Bosisto's Eucalyptus Oil continued to increase with interest being fostered through international exhibitions. Between 1854 and 1891 Bosisto's Eucalyptus Oil was exhibited and was awarded prizes in 17 international exhibitions.

At the Victorian Exhibition of 1861, Bosisto displayed 28 samples of oil from different plants, mainly eucalypts. Medals won at other international exhibitions are shown below :

1862	London Exhibition	Bronze Medal
1863	London Society of Arts	Silver Medal
1865	Dublin International Exhibition	Bronze Medal
1873	London Annual International Exhibition	Gilt Medal
1873	Vienna International Exhibition	Bronze Medal
1875	Melbourne International Exhibition	2 Silver Medals
1876	Philadelphia International Exhibition	Bronze Medal
1878	Paris International Exhibition	2 Bronze Medals
1879	Sydney International Exhibition	1 Silver, 1 Bronze Medal
1880	Melbourne International Exhibition	Bronze Medal
1883	Amsterdam International Colonial Exhibition	2 Gold, 1 Silver Medal
1883	Calcutta International Exhibition	3 Silver, 1 Bronze Medal
1886	London Colonial and Indian Exhibition	5 Bronze Medals
1887	Adelaide Jubilee International Exhibition	Bronze Medal

Sales were brisk following a lively promotion campaign. Bosisto produced an elaborate new label and a thousand circulars attesting to the powerful properties of Oil of Eucalyptus for "arts, manufacturers, medicine and sanitary purposes" which were distributed throughout the colonies and in Europe.

A very popular use at this time and during the influenza epidemic of 1918-19 was the addition of two or three drops of eucalyptus oil on to a teaspoon of sugar. The mixture was slowly dissolved in the mouth.

Consumer comments

> "I am a great user of your eucalyptus oil. We are fourth-generation users. My grandmother used to give us two or three drops on a teaspoon with sugar for sore throats, colds or flu."
>
> J.A. Vic

> "Having used the oil most of my life I can vouch for it. Father, I remember in childhood, as soon as he got a cold, 4 drops on a teaspoon of sugar fixed him. I still do it."
>
> D.C. Vic

Note: The above use is no longer permitted to avoid the possibility of over-dosing and accidental poisoning.

By the turn of the century oil was being exported to the United Kingdom, Germany, USA, Canada, South Africa, India, China, New Zealand and several countries in the Far East.

Bosisto's other eucalyptus products

In addition to the oil itself, Bosisto produced cigarettes of *Eucalyptus globulus* which were recommended for bronchial and asthmatic problems and for their disinfectant and antiseptic properties. They could be bought with or without tobacco. His Red Gum Lozenges were highly recommended for public speakers and singers.

Bosisto also had a profitable line in Syrup of Red Gum for bowel complaints which he claimed was very soothing. Another product was 'Liquor Eucalypti Globuli' (the fever and ague remedy) which was claimed to counteract malaria without any deleterious effect on the nervous system.

Medical journal reports in the 1880s

Although Bosisto's claims may appear exaggerated, they were in line with the medical research at that time. *The Lancet* in 1880 recommended surgical dressing gauze be dipped in a solution of eucalyptus oil, alcohol and water. *The British Medical Journal* in 1882 recommended eucalyptus oil vapour as a substitute for carbolic spray.

An article in *The Practitioner* May, 1885, recounted that of 220 cases of typhoid fever treated with eucalyptus oil during 18 months, only four patients had died.

Dr J H Mussen of Philadelphia presented a paper which was published in *The Therapeutic Gazette* in July 1886 "on the value of Oil of Eucalyptus in some malarial afflictions". He found the oil had benefit but the results from large doses of quinine were better.

The Lancet and *Medical Times* published reports stating that diphtheria had been treated successfully with eucalyptus oil and that a mixture of eucalyptus oil and olive oil had proved to be a good liniment for rheumatism and sciatica.

By 1900, Bosisto's Eucalyptus Oil was well established and the firm was able to supply the world market with substantial quantities of various types of high-grade oils.

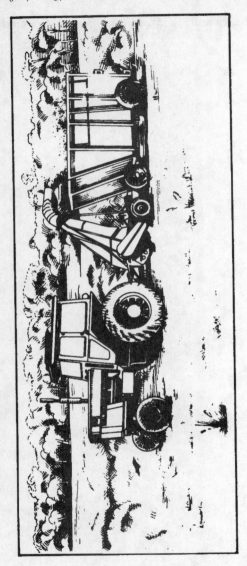

Modern harvester cutting Blue Mallee for Bosisto's Eucalyptus Oil.

Australian
Production

Early production

The production of eucalyptus oil in the 1880's was often carried out by Aborigines and by erstwhile miners as the goldfields petered out. It was hard work and very labour-intensive. The virgin scrub was cut by hand with slashers and special sickles.

The eucalyptus branches and leaves were collected and carted by wagon to the distillery where the freshly cut material was dumped into vertical iron stills set into the ground below wagon level for easy filling. After steam had carried over the volatile oil, the spent leaves and stick were hoisted out by derrick and dumped on the fire, whose rising column of smoke was a constant landmark.

The old distilleries were somehow kept going by pieces of wire, bits of tin, lumps of clay and the infinite resourcefulness of the true bush workman whose ramshackle buildings were made of hand-hewn posts and roofed with branches of nearby trees.

Things changed after World War II. The old worker gave way to the younger generation who would no longer accept the same living conditions that had prevailed in the past.

By about 1950 the cost of producing eucalyptus oil in Australia had increased so much the oil could no longer compete against Spanish and Portuguese oils on international markets.

The labour cost however, was not the only cause of the decline. After World War II there was a strong demand for Australian wheat and this entailed drastic destruction of stands of high-quality eucalyptus species. Improved wheat strains and modern farming machinery allowed wheat to be grown successfully on land formerly suited only for eucalyptus. The class-conscious prosperous Australian wheat farmers have always been inclined to look on eucalyptus oil production as a low-grade occupation. Wheat growing appeared to be more profitable than eucalyptus oil production.

Australia dominated the world eucalyptus oil market for over 80 years. Regretfully, Australia's market share then declined.

Australian production on the increase

Happily the downward trend is now being reversed – at least for medicinal oils. Advances in science and technology have been combined to modernise the industry.

By introducing mechanical harvesting and new distillation equipment, the cost of production has been reduced greatly. This, together with the natural advantages Australia has in growing stands of eucalypts with high quality pharmaceutical oils, has given the industry an opportunity to again become the dominant supplier in world trade.

WA salinity may boost eucalyptus oil production

Western Australia has an estimated 1.8 million hectares of farmland (10 per cent of the productive area) already salt-affected to some extent and this area could double in the next 15 – 25 years and then double again. Over a third of the state's divertible water resources is brackish or saline and a further 16 per cent is of marginal quality.

Salinity also poses a major threat to natural diversity (biological and physical), rural towns, capital infrastructure, tourism and recreation areas and the ability to support new export industries.

The fundamental cause of salinity is the replacement of perennial, deep-rooted native vegetation with the annual crops and pastures used in agriculture. Annual crops and pastures do not use as much of the incoming rainfall as did the native vegetation (even in low rainfall areas). This unused water either runs off or infiltrates beyond the root zone and accumulates as ground water.

As the ground waters rise, salts that have accumulated in the subsoil for thousands of years are brought close to the surface reducing plant vigour and eventually causing death of the plant.*

Salinity - a situation statement for Western Australia by the CEO's of the WA Departments of Agriculture, Conservation and Land Management, Environmental Protection and the Water and Rivers Commission November 1996).

To help remedy this huge dry land salinity disaster in the wheatbelt, WA government departments, farmers, universities and industry have combined to investigate the possibility of planting millions of deep-rooted oil 'mallee' trees to soak up the excess water and lower the water table.

A second objective of the study is to see if a viable eucalyptus oil distillery can be established which would provide farmers with an on-going income.

Already 12 million trees have been planted. They are growing very well and early indications are they are achieving their goals.

'Blue mallee' trees have produced good oil yields and five or six WA mallee species identified by the Department of Conservation and Land Management as high eucalyptus oil producers, have also done well.

The growers Oil Mallee Association aims to plant 500 million oil-producing eucalypts in the next 20 years, if the current trials are successful.

Felton Grimwade & Bickford is assisting with this important land care program and the company has agreed to purchase the entire quantity of medicinal eucalyptus oil produced in WA for at least the first three years of commercial operation.

Main eucalyptus species presently exploited

Eucalyptus polybractea, commonly known as 'blue mallee', is a small mallee-type tree. It grows only in natural stands in the districts north and north-west of Bendigo in Victoria and in the West Wyalong area in New South Wales.

The yield of oil from the leaves and terminal branchlets varies between 1.5 and 2.5 per cent.

The crude oil is high in cineole and usually assays at between 80 and 88 per cent.

Eucalyptus radiata var. australiana, commonly known as 'narrow-leaved peppermint', is a medium sized tree with fibrous bark. It occurs in extensive areas in Victoria and the south coast districts and southern highlands of New South Wales.

The yield of oil from the leaves and terminal branchlets averages between 2.5 and 3.5 per cent.

The crude oil has a cineole content of 65-70 per cent and has a very refreshing aroma.

Production has fallen as costs have become too high. The leaves cannot be mechanically harvested in the same way as *E. polybractea*.

Eucalyptus globulus was discovered in Tasmania in 1792 by Labillardiere and is commonly known as the 'Tasmanian blue gum'. No eucalypt has received so much attention from botanists and chemists as this species.

It has been cultivated in all parts of the world and the eucalyptus oil from *E. globulus* is the best known and most used of all eucalyptus oils. While it was distilled in Tasmania in 1880, it is no longer produced in Australia, having been replaced by higher yielding and better quality oils from other species.

The yield of oil from the leaves and branchlets averages from 0.75 to 1.25 per cent.

The cineole content is between 60 – 70 per cent and since in many instances the properties of the crude oil do not meet the specifications of most pharmacopoeias, the oil has to be treated to increase the cineole content.

Eucalyptus citriodora, commonly known as the 'lemon-scented gum'. Recently it underwent a name change and is now called *Corymbia*. A large tree often reaching a great height with a smooth whitish pale pink bark. Readily identified by the fragrant 'citronella-like' odour of the crushed leaves, it grows extensively in Queensland in natural stands.

The yield of oil from the leaves and terminal branchlets from forest trees varies from 0.5 to 0.75 per cent and from cultivated trees up to two per cent.

The principal constituent of the oil is citronellal and the oil is used for industrial and perfumery purposes. Large quantities of oil were once distilled in Queensland. However, Brazil and China, which have extensive plantations, now produce almost all the oil from this species.

Production today

Bosisto's 'Parrot' Brand Eucalyptus Oil is produced from 5000 hectares of unique natural forest in the Inglewood and Wedderburn districts of central Victoria.

Most of the oil produced is derived from 'blue mallee' *(E. polybractea)* known to produce the most potent medicinal oil from all of the hundreds of eucalyptus species tested.

The blue mallee tree only grows to waist height before being harvested every two years. The mallee roots are hundreds of years old and are ever ready to send up new growth after each harvest.

The land on which 'blue mallee' has been regularly cut every two years has the purest and healthiest stands. Some areas have been harvested for 100 years with no evidence of damage to the trees. It appears the trees thrive under these conditions which are not unlike the regular burning off of the old wood by Aborigines long before white man discovered Australia.

Considerable improvement has been made in recent years in the harvesting, materials handling and distillation of 'blue mallee'. While not as picturesque as the old superseded methods, three men can now produce the same quantity of oil as 100 men did in the early days.

Harvesting

'Blue mallee' is the only major oil producing species which can be mechanically harvested. As the species is confined to Australia, it enables Bosisto's Eucalyptus Oil to compete against competitors with low labour costs.

The 'blue mallee' is cut by a harvester a few centimetres from the ground. The cut material is thrown up a chute directly into a mobile still which is towed behind. Once the mobile still is filled with about three tonnes of leaf, it is uncoupled and another still attached. When two or three stills are filled a second trailer tows the stills to the distillery.

Distillation

After the mobile stills enter the distillery, lids are placed on them and clamped into position to ensure a good seal. Steam is connected at the base of the stills and the steam vaporises the oil. The vapours are carried over into modern stainless steel condensers where they are condensed into a mixture of oil and water.

The mixture is then collected in a receiver where separation takes place. The eucalyptus oil being lighter floats to the surface and is decanted off. The yield of oil varies but averages about one per cent of the biomass harvested.

It takes 5kg (12lb) of leaf and twigs to produce enough oil for a 50mL bottle.

The oil is later redistilled to remove any impurities. No artificial additives, aromas or flavourings are used. No pesticides or fertilisers are used.

By-product a valuable garden mulch

After distillation, the lids are lifted and the mobile stills are towed out for emptying of the spent leaves and twigs. This by-product meets all the criteria of a first-class mulch and ground cover.

The mulch is weed free and non-toxic to animals and plants. It suppresses weed growth and reduces the need for watering. It stays in place even in very high winds. Landscape architects and home gardeners particularly like its natural appearance and bushland fragrance. After two or three years the mulch breaks down into organic humus.

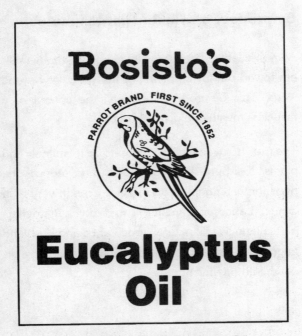

Bosisto's Parrot Brand Eucalyptus Oil.

Bosisto's 'Parrot' Brand Eucalyptus Oil

Bosisto's 'Parrot' Brand Eucalyptus Oil has been first in eucalyptus oil since 1852. Over the years the knowledge and experience gained has been incorporated into the final product.

Bosisto's 'Parrot' Brand Eucalyptus Oil is a 100 per cent pure premium quality pharmaceutical grade eucalyptus oil. It is a natural steam-distilled oil. The crude oil is later redistilled to remove any impurities and to improve the keeping qualities of the oil. It is an entirely natural organic product.

Bosisto's 'Parrot' Brand Eucalyptus Oil has one of the most characteristic odours of the eucalyptus oils. It is strong and pronounced. When first smelled, one notices a roundness of odour, a fullness which is then penetrated by the characteristic smell of cineole. As the oil evaporates there is left a spicy residual note reminiscent of nutmeg.

Other eucalyptus oils are camphoraceus and medicinal but do not have the depth and woodiness of the best eucalyptus oil Their odour is light and indefinite.

You can easily compare the difference between Bosisto's 'Parrot' Brand Eucalyptus Oil and other eucalyptus oil. Simply put, a couple of drops of oil on the back of each hand. You will be able to smell the difference in fragrance and how long the fragrance lasts.

Consumer Comments

"You are probably wondering what I use Bosisto's Eucalyptus Oil for.

I have several candle burners in five rooms for cigarette smoke, mildew, dampness and for a deodoriser.

Mixing your oil with water in a spray bottle, to spray inside my boys smelly shoes, wardrobes, along all sliding windows for the bugs that do get through the fly screens and doors, my dog and his bed, wiping over our bed heads, spraying onto silk flowers and into the bag of my vacuum cleaner, all my floors and veneer furniture and all your hints from your booklet with it.

My son is asthmatic and loves having his burner on all night and his pillows, furniture, hankies are sprayed with the oil and his clothes are washed with a few drops of the oil.

As we live on a one-acre property it is great to use for the saddles, cleaning up after floods, cleaning our garbage bin as we get once a week pick up and you can imagine the smell and maggots and I find it is a great repellent for snails and bugs. I mix a few drops in a Chinese container with water and it keeps snails, bugs and neighbours pets out of my gardens.

I could go on and on of how I use it, as I found the best purpose is that I do not have to worry about inhaling any poisonous chemicals and especially wearing a mask."

G.E. NSW

"I have been using your eucalyptus oil for all manner of things washing, foot baths, baths, bathing wounds, cleaning cupboards, floors etc. keeping away insects (and I don't think mice like it either!) in carpet cleaning and just to make rooms smell alive too!"

L.M. WA

"I use so much Bosisto's Eucalyptus Oil around my small place.

- *It removes the labels from bottles, plastic etc.*

- *It removes paint from my hands, drops on floors, smears on walls and a few weeks ago it was used to remove paint from the hair of a well-loved dog who had tried to help the family paint the house. It was painless, quick and certainly made him smell well for a while.*

- *More recently I used it to remove vast quantities of Blue Tack from a bedroom wall where many posters had been stuck on the walls. A scraper removed the larger lumps of Blue Tack and a large piece of cotton wool soaked in Bosisto's Eucalyptus*

Oil was used to soak the remains and then using a larger stiff tooth brush and more eucalyptus and plenty of elbow grease. Not a sign remains on the beautifully clean walls and the room smells so fresh.

- It is essential in the bathroom – toilet area and keeps my "under-the-sink" cupboard space presentable.

- Many years ago my grandfather always rubbed his back with eucalyptus before donning his thick, red-flannel waist belt at the beginning of winter. He renewed it every week after his weekly bath (we only had tanks) before wrapping himself into a fresh red-flannel belt."

J.D. Vic

"We use Bosisto's Eucalyptus for getting spots off clothes, the carpet and the dog! My grotty brother has the rotten habit of sleeping with parts of his beloved motorbike which miraculously find their way into his bedroom, his clothes, his cupboard, the carpet and even into the lounge room.

*The dog, which trails him everywhere,
usually ends up covered in grease too, so
some eucalyptus is dropped into his wash as
well.*

*Mum also has to dose my brother up with
eucalyptus as he goes out riding rain, hail or
shine. She makes him inhale it and
sometimes rubs his chest with it. What a
wimp! It's a wonder he doesn't just eat gum
leaves!!"*

J.L. Vic

The 100 per cent pure premium quality
pharmaceutical grade eucalyptus oil is available in
glass bottles of 50mL, 100mL and 200mL from the
Health and Beauty section of supermarkets and
pharmacies. Special plastic containers in one and four
litres are available directly from the manufacturer.

Bosisto's 'Parrot' Brand Eucalyptus Spray

Bosisto's 'Parrot' Brand Eucalyptus Spray is a
relatively recent addition to the range and it
complements the use of Bosisto's 'Parrot' Brand
Eucalyptus Oil.

Bosisto's 'Parrot' Brand Eucalyptus Spray is a high-quality pharmaceutical grade eucalyptus oil in an easy- to-use aerosol. It contains a special blend of Australian eucalyptus oils which are noted for their quality and fragrance. The fragrance is fresh and clean and there is no residual odour.

Bosisto's 'Parrot' Brand Eucalyptus Spray is a multi-use spray with a broad range of practical and worthwhile applications. It has the fresh, clean fragrance of the Australian bush.

Bosisto's 'Parrot' Brand Eucalyptus Spray is available in 200g cans from the Health and Beauty section of supermarkets and pharmacies.

Consumer Comments

> *"I have been using Bosisto's eucalyptus in some form all my life for so many different things. When it was brought out in a can it made it so much easier, as my husband has been quite ill with cancer and the treatment would make him quite nauseous, especially cooking smells. A quick spray through the house would keep the air fresh for him. I also use it as a laundry spray, toilet cleaner, disinfectant, antiseptic and goodness knows*

*what else. I even spray my little dog's kennel
and bedding with it to keep it free of fleas."*

N.W. Vic

*"I am very happy with your Eucalyptus
Spray. We used it for arthritis.*

*We were holidaying and had vandals paint
all our new car with red paint. We were very
upset. Then we asked everybody how could
we get it off. No-one knew so I suggested to
my husband what about our Eucalyptus
Spray and he said it is worth a try. We were
frightened to put it on paint work. But we
took all the paint off the tyres, wheelcaps and
lights and it was wonderful. It took every
trace of paint off. We have told everyone
what a wonderful job the spray did."*

M.S. Taree N.S.W

*"I suffer from severe allergies to any other
spray other than this wonderful all- purpose
spray"*

P.M. NSW

Uses of Bosisto's Eucalyptus Oil and Spray

Medicinal Uses

Head colds, influenza

You will get great relief from the following treatment. Pour 15 to 20 drops of Bosisto's 'Parrot' Brand Eucalyptus Oil in a bowl of steaming hot water and inhale, covering your head with a towel. To make it easier to breathe, sprinkle a few drops on your handkerchief. Freshen the sick room with Bosisto's Eucalyptus Spray.

Children's colds

Gently massage child's chest and back. For very young infants, mix the oil with an equal part of olive oil or other vegetable oil.

Consumer comments

> *"I have been using Bosisto's Eucalyptus Oil, especially on my handkerchief. This year I put it on my handkerchief and just inside the open end of the pillow. It was good at night times."*
>
> *I.O. Vic*

> *"I find Bosisto's Eucalyptus Spray useful for so many things in and around the home. It is particularly good at night, making it much easier to breathe when I have sinus."*
>
> *V.N. NSW*

"I found your Bosisto's Eucalyptus Oil very effective for my baby as an after-bath rub on her chest, particularly as she was having some phlegm. I noticed she breathed more freely after a few applications."

L.M. Malaysia

Muscular aches and pains

You will obtain soothing relief from the muscular aches and pains of arthritis, rheumatism, fibrositis, sprained tendons and ligaments, strained, bruised, stiff and sore muscles by gently massaging Bosisto's Eucalyptus Oil or Spray into affected areas until a warm glow is felt. Repeat at intervals until the pain or swelling disappears.

Consumer comments

"During the night I could not get out of bed because of severe cramp pains in my right leg. I rubbed Bosisto's Eucalyptus Oil into the calf and in a short time the pain completely disappeared."

R. M. Vic

"I have arthritis in my neck and spine which at times I can hardly bear the headaches and the only real relief I get is from rubbing your eucalyptus oil."

Y.F. Vic

"I should like to tell you of the benefit of the use of your eucalyptus oil, which I use on arthritic knees and ankles. I find that I have less pain in the joints and also less swelling from fluid retention in the joints. There was a great tendency for the locking of joints, which is most painful. Most of this has been eased with several months of treatment."

D.D. SA

"My daughter has a very bad back and the spray is the only thing to help her."

R.M. Qld

"Bosisto's Eucalyptus Spray provided great relief to severe back pain experienced by my great aunt."

C.M. NSW

"My husband is a courier and runs up and down a lot of steps and the old knees and muscles ached. He has found Bosisto's Eucalyptus Spray was very good. He even carried a can in the car."

G.W. NSW

Training oil

A warming, soothing liniment that helps get muscles loosened and ready to go. Massage Bosisto's Eucalyptus Oil into muscles until a warm glow is felt. If the 'bite' is too strong, mix oil with baby oil or any vegetable oil.

Asthma

Eliminating house dust mites reduces the risk of asthma. Bosisto's Eucalyptus Spray sprayed in the room and Bosisto's Eucalyptus Oil in the laundry wash have been shown to be highly effective in controlling house dust mites and their allergens.

See Hints and Recipes. Dust Mite Control Program (page 87)

Consumer comments

> "Bosisto's Eucalyptus Oil when laundering
> bedding has produced a marked reduction in
> asthma symptoms in our household."
>
> *J.M. New Zealand*

> "We have found another use for the spray –
> we keep it handy in the bathroom. My
> husband is asthmatic and when he has a
> 'tight' chest makes sure when he showers the
> bathroom is full of steam and the spray in the
> steam seems to help."
>
> *L.L. SA*

> "Bosisto's Eucalyptus Spray is a very
> effective product in the house, deodorising,
> disinfecting and it has no effect on my
> husband who is asthmatic and allergic to
> many sprays."
>
> *S.M. NSW*

"Your wonderful product called Bosisto's Eucalyptus Spray 'Parrot' Brand. I'm a mother of two daughters that suffer from asthma and are allergic to every room freshener with the exception of yours."

R.M. NSW

Insect bites

You can get quick relief from the pain of insect bites by applying Bosisto's Eucalyptus Oil or Spray on to sore and swollen areas. Repeat if necessary.

Mouthwash

For a refreshing mouthwash place two drops of oil on toothpaste when cleaning teeth or add a few drops of oil to a glass of water and gargle.

Bath and foot bath

Adding one or two teaspoons of Bosisto's Eucalyptus Oil to bath water is very invigorating and gives a feeling of well-being. A teaspoon of oil in a foot bath gives excellent relief.

Consumers Comments

> *"I regularly soak in the bath with some oil as*
> *I have back, knee and shoulder disorders*
> *and I find this is beneficial."*

L.McN. NSW

> *"My idea of heaven is a nightly bath to which*
> *is added about one-third of a 50mL bottle of*
> *Bosisto's Eucalyptus Oil."*

J.H. Vic

Vaporiser-Humidifier

You will get relief from many respiratory ailments if you add a few drops of Bosisto's Eucalyptus Oil to your steam vaporiser. The air will smell fresher too.

Scalp Massage

Rub a few drops of oil into scalp or add to shampoo to stimulate blood flow to hair roots.

Consumer comments

"Bosisto's Eucalyptus Oil is very good for an itchy scalp. I rub it well into my scalp in the evening, leave it overnight and wash thoroughly next morning."

Mrs M. Vic

"Bosisto's 'Parrot' Brand Eucalyptus Oil is very well known to me as I have been using it for various purposes for years – I always add a few drops to the water when washing combs and hair brushes as it thoroughly cleanses and disinfects them."

M.S. Vic

Sauna

Give your sauna a fresh, clean, country smell by adding some Bosisto's Eucalyptus Oil to water for splashing on hot stones or around sauna. You will find it helps clear your head and makes breathing easier.

See Hints and Recipes – Use in saunas (page 79)

Air freshener

Bosisto's Eucalyptus Spray has the pure fresh fragrance of the Australian bush. It's the perfect natural air freshener. Its ideal for the toilet, bathroom and sick room and for clearing stale smoke fumes.

Insect repellent

Bosisto's Eucalyptus Spray is a good mosquito repellent. To prolong protection, rub on a mixture of eucalyptus oil and vegetable or baby oil.

Consumer comments

"Bosisto's 'Parrot' Brand Eucalyptus Spray is very useful against the multifarious mosquitoes and other such wildlife which challenge comfortable living in the tropics."

D.D. Qld

"I have a small cupboard in which is stored my hot water heater and it was a breeding ground for hundreds of cockroaches. Since placing a cloth sprinkled with a few drops of Eucalyptus Oil on it once a week I have not

*seen one cockroach. I have now placed a
small piece of cloth, as above, under my
refrigerator and have no doubt my place will
be 'cockroach free' this summer. Added to
this, a pleasant fragrance is a bonus. Thanks
for an excellent product."*

D.N. NSW

Household Uses

Spot and stain remover

You will find it easy to remove oil soluble grease and
grass marks, spots and stains from clothes, carpets and
fabric with a cloth moistened with Bosisto's Eucalyptus
Oil. Where possible, put an absorbent cloth under the
stained area. By brushing towards the centre of the
mark you will prevent the formation of a ring. Bosisto's
Eucalyptus Oil is harmless to material and does not
stain or smear.

Bosisto's Eucalyptus Spray is also wonderful for
getting out stubborn stains and grease marks on
carpets, clothes and fabrics. It is ideal on carpets.
Simply spray and wipe. The carpet stays dry. You can
walk on it immediately and there is no resoiling.

Consumer comments

> *"I use a great deal of Bosisto's Eucalyptus Oil to remove grease stains from my family's clothes. My youngest daughter works for McDonald's and has numerous grease stains from cooking oil and I have found your eucalyptus oil to be the only successful product to remove the grease. The bottled oil I find is excellent but the spray can is perfect."*
>
> K. McL NSW

> *"I use your eucalyptus oil to remove stains on my clothing and to clean my limited collection of teddy bears."*
>
> C.L. Singapore

> *"I am self-employed in the car detailing industry and use your product Bosisto's Eucalyptus Oil to remove oil, grease, chewing gum and other stubborn stains from upholstery and carpets. I find your oil an excellent product."*
>
> R.M. Tas

Adhesive labels

Bosisto's Eucalyptus Oil or Spray is excellent for removing adhesive labels from articles without damage or abrasion to most articles. As a precaution, test on unseen area first. Adhesive bandages and sticking plaster dampened with oil will lift off easily and painlessly.

Ballpoint ink marks

You can quickly take out ballpoint ink marks from clothes, shoes and furnishings with Bosisto's Eucalyptus Oil or Spray

Consumer comments

> *"Bosisto's 'Parrot' Brand Eucalyptus Spray is used in the book shop to remove biro pen marks and to freshen up stock."*
>
> *M.D. Tas*

Chewing gum

Bosisto's Eucalyptus Oil is excellent for removing chewing gum from hair, clothes and shoes.

Hand and skin cleaner

Excellent for cleaning hands and skin of unpleasant smells. Removes grease and paint. Wash with Bosisto's Eucalyptus Oil or rub with cloth moistened with oil and then with soap and water as usual.

Washing clothes, especially work clothes and nappies

Clean and freshen by adding a teaspoonful or two of Bosisto's Eucalyptus Oil to each load of wash. Ideal for overalls, sportswear, socks and nappies.

Consumer comments

> "My husband works on the Shire Council as a loader operator and he wears white combination overalls which get very dirty and greasy. The only way I can get the grease out is with Bosisto's Eucalyptus. I use one teaspoonful added to the washing water."
>
> F.S. NSW

*"I use Bosisto's Eucalyptus Oil for washing
and soaking my son's overalls to help clean
the grease off them."*

B.H. Vic

Laundry pre-wash

Bosisto's Eucalyptus Spray is marvellous for taking out
grease marks on clothes. Spray soiled areas, leave a
minute then wash in normal manner.

Consumer comments

*"I work in a childcare centre and we used
your Bosisto's Eucalyptus Oil in the centre
and would proclaim its uses as a pre-wash
spotter to remove the daily grime of paint
and play etc."*

P.S. NSW

Carpet cleaner

Stains and grease marks are easy to get out of carpets
with Bosisto's Eucalyptus Spray. Just spray the spots
and stains and wipe them away with a clean absorbent
cloth. Your carpet stays dry and ready for use.

Consumer comments

"We built a lovely new house, got the carpet down and when we were shifting in the furniture some **tar** was stuck to a shoe off the new drive and walked inside all the way upstairs. I could have cried when I saw these sticky black spots on my pale rye carpet.

I found your Eucalyptus Spray – it worked – the tar just lifted off and I was thrilled.

I couldn't believe it – what a life saver."

G.D. Vic

General Cleaning

Add a teaspoon of Bosisto's Eucalyptus Oil to the water when washing floors. It's great for cleaning and deodorising and it smells good too.

Bosisto's Eucalyptus Oil and Spray cleans grease from glass, enamel and other hard surfaces. It is ideal for cleaning hard to remove marks from white boards.

Consumer comments

"Bosisto's Eucalyptus Oil does a wonderful job cleaning the jarrah floor boards."

W.F. NT

"I had tried removing black scuff marks from my kitchen floor to no avail. I was beginning to despair when I found Bosisto's Eucalyptus Spray. I sprayed it on the marks, waited a few seconds then rubbed the marks away like magic. Thanks for this wonderful Australian product."

J.W. Vic

"Only recently have I discovered the marvellous product Bosisto's Eucalyptus Oil and I am wondering why it is such a well-kept secret. I use your product for practically every cleaning job in the home and office, finding that my other cleaners are now redundant and expensive."

E.D. Vic

> *"Your Eucalyptus Oil is used in our office on
> the white board. It cleans writing that has
> been on the board for a while and the office
> always smells fresh, especially in the
> mornings when we start work."*

> H.B. Qld

Telephone

Bosisto's Eucalyptus Oil is a great way to clean and disinfect your telephone. Simply wipe with a cloth dampened with the oil.

Toilet

Freshen and deodorise with Bosisto's Eucalyptus Spray. A teaspoon of Bosisto's Eucalyptus Oil in toilets or drains is a good disinfectant, cleaner and deodoriser.

Consumer comments

> *"I have used Bosisto's Eucalyptus for many
> years. I also use it in the toilet in a jar which
> is covered with a cloth every few days."*

> M.H. Vic

"Bosisto's Eucalyptus Spray was recommended by a stoma patient in the magazine Ostomy. We have found that the highly artificially perfumed sprays do not deodorise toilets but 'the Parrot' does."

B.O. Qld

Plastic and vinyl

Bosisto's Eucalyptus Oil is excellent for cleaning ink, printing ink, carbon and other marks off most plastic and vinyl. Test on unseen area first to ensure it will not affect plastic surface.

Leather cleaner

Wet a clean cloth and add a few drops of Bosisto's Eucalyptus Oil. Wipe over marked area. It does not harm the leather but always use a damp cloth, or test a patch on an unseen part.

Paint brushes

Oil paint brushes can be restored by soaking in eucalyptus oil

Consumer comments

"I am now washing my paint brushes in eucalyptus oil. It cleans them clean and now makes the use of this hot soap and water part of the cleaning process tolerable to me. Turps is illing – to nose, face and stomach and me."

B.H. Vic

Tar marks on paintwork of motor vehicles

You can easily remove tar marks by rubbing with a cloth moistened with Bosisto's Eucalyptus Oil. For large areas you can dilute one part of oil with four parts kerosene, petrol or vinegar or simply spray and wipe clean.

Car tyres

Spray around the rim of the tyre with Bosisto's Eucalyptus Spray to deter dogs from marking their territory around your car.

Hints *and* recipes

There are so many wonderful recipes we can make that are natural and effective. These take so little time in the busy world we live in and it becomes almost therapeutic, just making them. As with all essential oils, they are very powerful and must be treated with respect. If the recipe says two drops, then three drops will not make it better.

Always keep your oils out of the reach of little ones and if you are pregnant, avoid wearing essential oils on your body and seek advice from your therapist.

Animals' sense of smell is hundreds of times more powerful than our own, so do not let your sense of smell be a guide when making products for your pets.

If you have sensitive skin and are in doubt as to whether you can use them, always try a patch test on the inside of the arm.

If you are taking homoeopathic medicines, do not use any essential oil on your skin – at least for a couple of hours – or check with your therapist.

Hair Care

Hair consists of around 97 per cent protein, the remaining three per cent being moisture. Hair roots lie below the surface of the skin in the small sac-shaped glands known as follicles. The function of each follicle is to produce keratin, a protein substance. An oil gland supplies a coating to each strand of hair to protect moisture in that strand.

It is said our hair is our crowning glory and, with the constant abuse of chlorine, heat and exposure to the environment, we can still have a healthy and beautiful head of hair.

Hot oil treatment

Our hair loves to be pampered and nothing looks nicer than clean, healthy and shiny hair.

> 50 mL olive oil
> 5 mL Bosisto's Eucalyptus Oil

Blend the eucalyptus oil into the olive oil and pour into a plastic or strong glass bottle. Stand in very hot water for 10 minutes or so to warm the oil. Massage gently on to scalp and brush or comb through the hair. Wrap in a clean towel or put on a shower cap and leave on for around 15 minutes. Shampoo and condition.

Itchy scalp

> 50 mL of cider vinegar
> 5 mL Bosisto's Eucalyptus Oil
> 1 litre spring water

Mix all ingredients together, shake well and add this to the final rinse after shampooing.

Run it through the hair several times to ensure effective coverage.

Protein gel

This works like a face pack for the hair.

> 10 gm plain gelatine
> 300 mL mineral water
> 5 mL witch-hazel
> 10 drops Bosisto's Eucalyptus Oil

Mix the gelatine and water together until you have a smooth liquid. Stir and leave it until it forms a gel type substance, do not let it set. Now add the witch-hazel and eucalyptus oil; this will prevent it from becoming solid. Use as a hair pack, covering all of the hair. Leave on for 10 minutes, then rinse off thoroughly. Use weekly.

Flaky scalp

> Natural shampoo (see recipe)
> 5 mL Bosisto's Eucalyptus Oil
> 10 drops lavender oil
> 10 drops basil oil

Blend into shampoo base, use every other day. This helps to remove the build-up of dead skin cells and is gentle enough to be used two to three times weekly.

Hair-stimulating shampoo

> 100 mL base shampoo recipe
> 15 drops jojoba oil
> 10 drops carrot oil
> 20 drops Bosisto's Eucalyptus Oil
> 10 drops rosemary oil
> 10 drops lavender oil

Blend the ingredients together in a double saucepan to be sure they are dispersed.

Use once a week.

Hair-stimulating conditioner

> 5 mL jojoba oil
> 10 drops evening primrose oil
> 10 drops Bosisto's Eucalyptus Oil
> 5 drops palma rosa oil

Blend together and massage gently into the scalp. Leave on hair for an hour, shampoo off with special hair-stimulating shampoo.

Shampoo base

Pure soap flakes can be obtained from some health food shops and pharmacies.

Castile soap is also excellent and should be pure and white.

> 100 grams pure soap flakes or Castile soap
> finely grated
> 1 litre spring water

Simmer the water, add the soap flakes, stir until all the soap has dissolved. Cool and bottle in a plastic container. If the mixture appears too thick, a little more spring water can be added, or pop into a blender if the mixture appears a little lumpy.

Soapwort shampoo

If you can obtain some soapwort root from a herbalist or Chinese herbalist, ask them to give you the crushed root of the plant.

> 15 grams crushed soapwort root
> 1 litre spring water

Boil the water and pour it over the soapwort in a bowl. Leave to infuse for at least an hour and then filter it through a fine cloth or filter. Strain again and bottle. You may find you need a little more of the solution to clean the hair, but it does a great job, and is the original raw material of many soaps and cleaning properties of old.

Conditioner

This easy to make conditioner works very well. When purchasing the ingredients, ask for liquid lecithin.

> 50 mL liquid lecithin
> 50 mL almond oil
> 15 mL jojoba oil
> 5 grams shea or cocoa butter

In a double saucepan, mix all ingredients together, stir until well blended together. Bottle into a clean plastic bottle. Using plastic for shampoo and conditioners is for safety reasons in the bathroom.

Vinegar conditioner

Cider vinegar is a simple but effective conditioner and to this you can add your essential oils to leave the hair shiny and clean. Shake well before using.

> 50 mL cider vinegar
> 2 mL Bosistos Eucalyptus Oil
> 1 litre spring water

The following is a list of Essential Oils that can help repair and leave your hair in a healthy condition. You will notice eucalyptus and lavender oils are relevant in all conditions and type of hair, as these oils are gentle, effective and balancing.

Oils for normal hair

Essential Oils of Eucalyptus, Lavender, Rosemary and Geranium.
Vegetable Oils; Almond, Peach kernel and Evening Primrose.

Oils for dry hair

Essential Oils of Eucalyptus, Lavender, Parsley and Sandalwood.
Vegetable Oils; Sesame, Jojoba, Avocado and Sunflower.

Oils for oily hair

Essential Oils of Eucalyptus, Lavender, Basil, Sage and Thyme.
Vegetable Oils; Evening Primrose, Sesame and Peach Kernel.

Oils for fragile and damaged hair

Essential Oils of Eucalyptus, Lavender, Chamomile, Calendula and Clary Sage.
Vegetable Oils; Jojoba, Almond oil, Borage Seed and Peach Kernel.

Consumer comment

> *"I have suffered with loss of hair through a nervous condition and have been many years trying everything – even a specialist, only to be told there was nothing anybody could do. The other day somebody told me to use eucalyptus oil which I did. I just couldn't believe the results. I have hair coming all over my head. I apply it each night, in the morning wash it off and massage my head. I noticed my hair showing in three weeks.*

I just couldn't put it in words what it means to me, only just a big thank you."

R.B. SA

Face and Body Care

The skin reflects our inner and general health, provides a water-proof barrier and excretes water salts, is a heat regulator and is a physical barrier against damage to the inner organs – so don't we really owe it and ourselves some maintenance?

No matter what your skin type, the following steps for total skin care improvement are essential for both men and women:

- effective cleansing
- toning
- exfoliation
- moisturising/protecting
- nourishing/conditioning

When making recipes for your skin, test a little of the finished product on the back of your wrist. Leave for a couple of hours if you have sensitive skin, then wash off. If you are allergic to any of the ingredients, this will become red and angry, or itchy.

Always dilute essential oils and never use directly on to the skin – they are very powerful ingredients.

Facial treatments

Our face is like a book. All that has gone before us is imprinted in our eyes, our expressions and the lines that etch their way. If we are happy, the face always appears younger. So with a little help to clean and exfoliate, eliminate bacteria and have that appearance of youth. The following recipes should help.

Our skin is the largest organ of our bodies. It is constantly regenerating and being subjected to various chemicals, air conditioners and the heat of the sun. There is little difference between male and female skin, so these formulas are well suited to both men and women.

Cleansing cream

100ml almond oil

125 grams ground almonds

50 mL witch-hazel

50 mL spring water

10 drops Bosisto's Eucalyptus Oil

5 drops lemon oil

Place all ingredients into a blender and mix for a couple of minutes until a paste has formed. Store in a clean, dark bottle out of direct sunlight. Use over a couple of weeks; it can be stored in the fridge for a longer life.

Soap cleanser

50 mL base soap shampoo base

50 mL liquid lecithin

20 mL witch-hazel

10 drops Bosisto's Eucalyptus Oil

5 drops lemon oil

2 drops lavender oil

Blend all ingredients together. Bottle in a clean bottle. When ready to use, pour a small amount into the palm of the hand and wash face and body, avoiding the eyes. Rinse off with warm water.

Facial scrub

These are effective if used once weekly. Make sure the almonds are finely ground to avoid sharp bits on your face.

> 1 teaspoonful of finely ground almonds
> (or a teaspoonful of cinnamon powder can be
> substituted for ground almonds)
> 1 teaspoonful oatflakes
> teaspoonful witch-hazel
> 3 drops of Bosisto's Eucalyptus Oil

Blend the witch-hazel and eucalyptus oil together, then add almonds and oatflakes, add a little water if mixture is very dry, in a circular motion gently apply the scrub, wash off with warm water. This can be used one to two times weekly.

Quick and easy scrub

> 1 teaspoonful finely ground almonds
> teaspoonful sweet almond oil
> 2 drops Bosisto's Eucalyptus Oil

Blend all ingredients together, massage over face, avoiding the eye area.

Leave on for 30 seconds; wash off with warm water.

Face masks

A face mask can greatly improve the condition of your skin. A mask can soothe inflammation, remove dirt and grime, prevent outbreaks and help exfoliate the outer layer of dead skin cells.

Fruit and vegetables can make a great mask, so if you have a very ripe avocado or some strawberries, don't throw them away. Mash them up, add a little rose water and a drop or two of eucalyptus and lavender oil, pat over the face and leave on for 10 minutes. Rinse off with warm water and moisturise. As easy as that!

Cooling mask

> 20 grams aloe vera gel
> 3 drops Bosisto's Eucalyptus Oil
> 1 drop carrot oil

Blend all ingredients together, keep in an airtight glass jar. Apply with clean fingertips, thickly over the face and neck. Leave on for five-10 minutes and rinse off with warm water.

A variation of this can be made with cucumber. Blend cucumber in blender and place in refrigerator until very cold. Stir in three drops eucalyptus oil and one drop carrot oil. Pack over face thickly, leave for 20 minutes, rinse off.

Clay is an ideal base for face masks and can be obtained easily from aromatherapy outlets. If you find you just can't find any, substitute cornflour, oats or rice flour. They also make great masks.

Revitalising clay mask

> 20 grams white or green clay powder
> 10 grams brewer's yeast
> 5 mL jojoba oil
> 10 mL water
> 3 drops Bosisto's Eucalyptus Oil
> 1 drop chamomile oil

Blend clay, oil and water, add essential oils. Apply over the face and allow to dry. Rinse off with warm water, apply a little jojoba oil after rinse. Do not store.

Facial tonics and astringents

A facial tonic can help the circulation, reduce the oily sections of the face and help to refine the pores. They are best used after facial cleansing or a facial scrub.

Skin tonic

> 100 mL rosewater.
> 5 drops Bosisto's Eucalyptus Oil
> 1 drop sandalwood oil

Blend all ingredients together. If you do not have any rosewater, make up a chamomile infusion, 1 tea bag to 100 mL distilled water. Shake before use. Both of these recipes will soothe inflamed skin, as well as toning it.

Astringent

> 75 mL rosewater or chamomile water.
> 25 mL witch-hazel water.
> 5 mL green tea (pour hot water on tea bag, squeeze 1 teaspoonful liquid)
> 6 drops Bosisto's Eucalyptus Oil
> 4 drops grapefruit oil

Blend all ingredients together. Shake before use. Apply after cleansing with a clean cotton ball.

Moisturising oils

Eucalyptus and essential oils really help to moisturise the skin. If you have oily skin – use grapeseed oil. For dry and dehydrated skin – sweet almond or peach kernel oil are ideal. Jojoba oil is a wonderful additive to any skin care regime and, although it is not an oil but a liquid wax, it helps to protect the skin and replenish lost moisture at the same time.

Rich moisturising oil

> 100 mL sweet almond oil
> 20 drops Bosisto's Eucalyptus Oil
> 10 drops sandalwood oil
> 10 drops patchouli oil
> 10 drops lavender oil

Blend all ingredients together; apply a little to the palm of the hand; warm by rubbing hands together; massage over face. A warm face flannel can be placed over the face if skin is extremely dry; this is called compressing.

Problem skin oil

> 50 mL grapeseed oil
> 30 mL evening primrose oil
> 20 mL jojoba oil
> 30 drops Bosisto's Eucalyptus Oil
> 20 drops lavender oil
> 10 drops tea tree oil

Blend all ingredients together and apply to face, keeping away from the eyes and do not apply to broken or irritated skin. Focus particularly on the problem area and always do a patch test first on the back of your wrist.

Blackhead treatment

> 50 mL spring water
> 20 mL witch-hazel
> 2 drops Bosisto's Eucalyptus Oil
> 2 drops cypress oil

Before applying this treatment, shake well.

Facial steaming is an ideal way to loosen blackheads. Fill a bowl with very hot water – be careful as steam can burn – add a teaspoonful of eucalyptus oil; place a towel over the head; allow the freshness of the steam to cleanse your skin and sharpen the mind. It is really fantastic if you have a sinus or a cold.

After steaming, apply the treatment by dabbing a little on to the area and steaming the face around once a week.

Moisturising cream

Some people prefer to use a cream and this is also ideal to wear under make-up for everyday use. Aqueous cream is a water-based cream and can be purchased from pharmacies and health shop outlets. If you cannot obtain it, a sorbolene base is also acceptable.

> 100 grams aqueous base
> 30 drops evening primrose oil
> 10 drops rose hip oil
> 10 drops Bosisto's Eucalyptus Oil
> 5 drops lavender oil
> 2 drops carrot oil

Blend all ingredients into base cream. If you require a thicker consistency add more aqueous base; for a lotion add a little distilled water. This should be placed in a sterile glass container and will last for several months. Use daily.

If you have a natural base lotion or cream at home, this can be an ideal medium to add to your essential oils. Always remember essential oils are very powerful so add the minimum amount and you can always add more later.

Consumer comment

"I have suffered from eczema and dermatitis for many years and have needed to wash everything in different products to reduce my redness and itching. It wasn't until I started using Bosisto's Eucalyptus Oil that my skin conditions have all but disappeared!!! I am so in love with your product that I wash everything in it. Not only is my skin back to near-normal but everything smells beautiful and clean. Now my skin looks great and it is all thanks to Bosisto's Eucalyptus Oil."

M.K Vic

Body wrap

If you have never experienced the wonderment of a body wrap, you could well be hooked once you have tried it. A body wrap is simple, cleansing, regenerating and refreshing and does wonders for a tired, worn- out body.

You will need a very large towel or sheet that can be wrapped around the body including the legs, you may feel a little like a 'mummy', but the effects are fantastic. If it is possible to warm the towel or sheet, you can get an added benefit from the body wrap and the heat will allow the oil to penetrate quickly.

If you happen to have a gorgeous partner, this recipe can be shared and made into a weekly or monthly ritual.

Regenerating body wrap

> 100 mL peach kernel oil
> 5 mL Bosisto's Eucalyptus Oil (1 teaspoonful)
> 20 drops rosemary oil

Blend ingredients together. Massage oil blend all over the body, avoiding the eye area. Include the neck, backs of hands and feet. Wrap the sheet or towel around you and relax for 20 minutes. Run a warm bath, take the phone off the hook and soak. This is ideal when you have to keep going but seem to have run out of energy.

Relaxing body wrap

100 mL sweet almond oil
30 drops lavender oil
20 drops bergamot oil
10 drops Bosisto's Eucalyptus Oil

Blend all together and use as a body wrap or as a rich moisturising oil. The lavender relaxes the mind, the bergamot brings a sense of happiness and the eucalyptus oil cleanses and relaxes sore, tired muscles.

Shower

Add a few drops of eucalyptus oil to a wet face cloth or sponge. Wash body as usual then briskly rub face cloth or sponge over the body. Close your eyes and inhale the beautiful aroma. Your body and mind will feel cleansed.

Two-minute revitaliser

Bosisto's produce a spray can of eucalyptus oil. If you are running short of time then simply spray eucalyptus over body, avoiding the eye area. Step into a warm shower or bath. The aroma of the oil clears the head, whilst the body benefits with a cleansing and regenerating effect.

Use in saunas

Bosisto's Eucalyptus Oil can be used in either wet or dry saunas or steam rooms. It clears the nose and makes breathing easier. It imparts a pleasant freshness to the air making a stay in a sauna room a pleasant experience. By using Bosisto's Eucalyptus Oil, the musty, wet, damp odour in wet areas can be greatly reduced.

Directions for use

Bosisto's Eucalyptus Oil should always be diluted with water before use. We recommend a 1.0 per cent solution to be used ie:

> 500mL water
> 5mL Bosisto's Eucalyptus Oil

Make up only enough solution for one or two days use. Do not store solution for longer than two days. Keep in a convenient sized plastic container with a trigger spray.

Before using always shake the container. Spray directly into the air or on to the walls. Do not spray directly onto hot coals or onto a radiant heat source.

Storage

i. Store in a **dry** place below 30C
ii. Keep containers tightly closed when stored
iii. Decant in a dry cool atmosphere

Warning

As eucalyptus oil is flammable, do not store the product or the made up spray solution near hot coals or a radiant heat source.

Safety

Bosisto's Eucalyptus Oil is perfectly safe to use provided the directions are followed.

After shave

Blend 80mL distilled water, 20mL vodka or gin and 50 drops of eucalyptus oil. Pat on after shaving. This will help to deter infected hair follicles.

Foot and Hand Care

Foot care

Our poor old feet take a lot of wear and tear. When our feet are tired, the whole body seems tired. Wearing shoes and socks daily stops the energy flow that begins in the feet and ends in the head region. This is one reason why a foot massage feels so good. One of the loveliest ways to do this at home regularly and enjoy the benefits, is with a good old-fashioned foot bath.

You will need:

> 1 large bowl – big enough to fit your feet into
> 6 marbles
> 1 clean face washer
> 10 mL Bosisto's Eucalyptus Oil

Fill the bowl with warm water and add the eucalyptus oil. Place the marbles in the bowl and cover with a face washer. Place one foot in and gently roll the marbles around with the sole of your foot – repeat process with other foot. Place both feet in after massage and allow to soak for 10 minutes. This is particularly good to do before cutting those tough toe nails; it softens them and allows dirt and grime to come away.

Chilblains

Consumer comment

> *"I use eucalyptus oil for the relief of chilblains. If you put some eucalyptus oil on cotton wool and dab it over your toes and heels night and morning it prevents itch and swelling."*

> *J.F. Vic*

Hand bath

Hands are a tell-tale sign of ageing, so pamper them now. This hand scrub can be performed weekly.

20 grams finely ground oats
teaspoonful cinnamon
30 drops Bosisto's Eucalyptus Oil
spring water to make a paste

Blend ingredients with water until you have a thick paste. Massage over backs of hands and palms. Have a bowl of warm water ready with one teaspoonful of eucalyptus oil. Rinse hands under tap and soak in bowl of water.

Lemon and eucalyptus hand bath

Never throw that lemon skin away before you give your hands and nails a scrub with it. The essential oil in the peel of the skin helps to remove dirt and stains off the hands. It also helps to remove yellow discolouration off the nails and tobacco stains from fingers. Fill a bowl with warm water and one teaspoonful of eucalyptus oil. Soak the lemon-treated hands in the eucalyptus and water for around two minutes. Wash and moisturise.

Nail bed treatment

Always seek medical advice if you have an infection or fungal irritation. To prevent these re-occurring the following treatment should help.

> 10 mL jojoba oil
> 20 drops Bosisto's Eucalyptus Oil
> 10 drops tea tree oil
> 10 drops lemon oil

Blend all together. With a cotton bud apply over nail and to the back of the nail. Do not dip cotton bud into blend as it will contaminate it very quickly. Leave this mixture on for as long as possible; use a pair of cotton gloves to keep it on longer. Soak off in a eucalyptus and water bowl.

Cuticle oil

> 10 mL olive oil
> 10 drops Bosisto's Eucalyptus Oil
> 6 drops grapefruit oil or lemon oil
> 5 drops geranium oil (optional)

Place a drop on the cuticle. With clean fingers massage into cuticle. Wash off and moisturise.

Colds, Aches and Allergies

Stuffy noses

A good old-fashioned inhalation can help clear the head when you have a stuffy nose or sinus. Headaches are often the result of a congested sinus region; this has the added benefit of giving you a facial steam at the same time.

Directions:

Fill a bowl with hot steamy water, and remember to be careful of the hot steam, place a towel over the head and inhale the aroma.

Use a wet handkerchief with a dash of eucalyptus oil and kept in a plastic sealed bag. Open the bag and inhale often.

A teaspoonful of aloe vera gel, five drops eucalyptus oil, gently wipe inside and around the nostril. This will soothe a sore, red and stuffy nose.

Consumer suggestion

"Á good recipe for colds and sore throats:

1 teaspoon Bosisto's Eucalyptus Oil

2 cups sugar

1 cup water

2 teaspoons honey

1 tablespoon white vinegar."

M.F. Vic

Muscular aches and pains

Now sport is supposed to be a healthy event, but sometimes we can overdo things and the results can be devastating. Protecting our muscles and joints can be a huge benefit later on. So before you embark on that marathon run, the following formula can be applied:

40 mL sweet almond oil

20 drops Bosisto's Eucalyptus Oil

10 drops rosemary oil

10 drops thyme oil

Blend these all together. Pour a little into the palms of the hands and warm. Rub over the legs, feet and whole body. Do this daily for at least a week before active sport.

If muscles and joints are sore, spray some eucalyptus oil on to area before and after sport.

Spray eucalyptus oil on to joints before bathing or showering. Soak in a warm bath with:

one cup of Lectric Soda (available at supermarkets) and one teaspoonful of eucalyptus oil. This is wonderful for arthritic people also.

Sprains, strains and bruises

> 50 mL olive oil
> 30 drops Bosisto's Eucalyptus Oil

Massage into affected areas until a warm feeling is experienced. Repeat this every couple of hours.

Dust Mite Control Program

Studies in the UK have shown that 80 per cent of asthmatic children were sensitive to house dust mites.

For asthmatics, lowering the dust mite population lowers the risk and the number of attacks.

House dust mite populations are highest around human and pet bedding. They like moist conditions, moderate temperatures and an ample supply of human and animal skin scales and other debris. They are actually too small to see, like the dark and love to live in feathers, blankets, mattresses, bed clothes, carpets and soft furnishings.

Yes, we all have them. Millions live in the cleanest of homes.

Bosisto's Eucalyptus Oil and Bosisto's Eucalyptus Spray have been shown to be highly effective in killing and controlling house dust mites. By using the spray in the room and the oil in the laundry wash combine to remove the allergens that cause asthmatic attacks.

Two-part control program

Part 1 – **Spray the room with Bosisto's Eucalyptus Spray.**
(By someone who is not asthmatic)

- All bedding and coverings which can be washed should be removed and set aside for washing.

- Open windows and doors before, during and immediately after spraying.

- Turn off all heaters, lights, electrical appliances and extinguish naked flames.

- Cover polished wood, acetate and acrylic plastic and delicate fabrics with plastic sheets.

- Hold Bosisto's Eucalyptus Spray about 20cm from surface and spray with a sweeping motion to thoroughly cover the area to be treated.

- Allow 15 seconds for each square metre. Each can will cover an area of 15-20 square metres.

- Spray mattresses, pillows, base cover, carpets, rugs, soft furnishings, curtains, soft toys and pet quarters.

- Leave for one to two hours.

- Vacuum all areas sprayed using a strong vacuum cleaner with a very fine filter bag (HEPA class filter or two-ply bag).

- Note. A special vacuum bag is essential otherwise the dust mite allergens will circulate in the air. It is better not to vacuum if a proper dust bag is not available. (Use a carpet sweeper instead).

- Repeat monthly. Vacuum as little as possible between treatments.

Precautions

- Bosisto's Eucalyptus Spray is flammable so do not spray or store near heat or open flames.

- Do not light or smoke cigarettes during treatment.

- Patch test a hidden area before spraying plastic surfaces or delicate fabrics and furnishings.

- Avoid continuous spray contact with skin.

Part 2 – **Wash bedding and coverings**

Wash all bedding and coverings, which are safe to wash in hot water (over 55C) on normal cycle to kill dust mites and remove allergens.

Use normal laundry detergent and add 10ml (two teaspoons) Bosisto's Eucalyptus Oil.

For woollen blankets and other sensitive fabrics unable to be washed in hot water, follow these steps.

Fill washing machine with lukewarm water (30C) to desired level.

Mix:

Bosisto's Eucalyptus Oil.	Parts	mL	mL	mL	%
	3	50	100	200	75
Sunlight Dishwashing Liquid.	1	18	35	70	25
Total Mix.		68	135	270	100

Check water capacity of your washing machine. (Note: Each brand and model take different volumes of water)

Some typical fill levels:

	Low	Medium	High
Water Capacity Litres	25	50	100
Add Mixture mL	68	135	270

(A standard double blanket is usually washed in approx. 50 litres of water)

- Mix briefly (one minute)
- Leave to soak for 30 minutes
- Wash on normal laundry cycle

A slightly higher percentage (almost 100 per cent) of mites are killed if the quantity of mixture is doubled or soaking time is extended to 60 minutes.

For Little People

New-born babies have very sensitive skin, so the use of essential oils should be very minimal for the first few months. One to two drops of eucalyptus oil diluted in a base oil of peach kernel or sweet almond oil is generally all that is needed.

Nappy rash

Fill a bowl with warm water and add one drop eucalyptus oil, one drop chamomile oil and one drop lavender oil. When you wash baby's bottom use a cotton ball and dip it into the water. When baby is dry mix a blend of the following.

> 50 ml aqueous or sorbolene cream
> 5 ml zinc cream
> 1 drop Bosisto's Eucalyptus Oil
> 1 drop chamomile oil
> 1 drop lavender oil

Mix these well together and apply to the bottom; repeat procedure each time you change the baby.

Cradle cap

    30 mL sweet almond oil
    1 drop eucalyptus oil
    1 drop geranium oil

Blend together, massage gently over baby's head avoiding the fontanelle. Repeat this daily until the scalp is clear.

Falls and scrapes

Dilute a couple of drops of eucalyptus oil in around a litre of cooled boiled water. With a cotton ball gently clean the affected area. Repeat this every couple of hours.

Little people's colds

    30 mL olive oil
    10 drops Bosisto's Eucalyptus Oil
    5 drops mandarin oil

Blend together and massage over chest and back.

Bug buster

Children can bring all sorts of things into the home, including other children's bugs. Always have a spray can of eucalyptus at hand to freshen the room, the bed and the toys.

Vaporising

If children are congested and feeling ill, a vaporiser can be a great help. Euky Bear vaporisers are available at pharmacies and can be hired for a day or a week. They are certainly not expensive to buy and not only are they ideal when people are congested, they also freshen up a stale home.

If you have an electric burner at home this can also freshen up those stale smells, but never use a candle burner as little ones can knock these over so easily, or the candle can ignite.

Take a hanky with a couple of drops of eucalyptus oil placed on it, pop it in between the pillow and pillowcase and the aroma will gently help the child to breathe easier.

Bruises, burns and cuts

To avoid infection always bathe the area and repeat this every couple of hours. Essential oils are great in their action to prevent infection, to soothe and promote healing. The most important thing to remember for children's skin is to dilute the oil. Burns respond very quickly to a combination of eucalyptus oil and lavender oil and will work even quicker if blended into cool green tea. Make up a strong solution of green tea, around 100 mL – add around 10 drops eucalyptus oil and 20 drops lavender oil, place in a spritzer, and spray the area that is burnt.

(Having lived in North Queensland when my children were young, I found this to be most effective on those occasions when a shoulder or back was left a little too long in the sun. – Cherie).

Growing pains

Little ones have many inexplicable pains, particularly as they grow so fast. When you are reassured it is simply part of growing the following blend will help the joints.

> 30 mL grapeseed oil
> 5 drops Bosisto's Eucalyptus Oil
> 5 drops geranium oil
> 5 drops lavender oil

Blend together. Gently massage with warmed hands the legs and knee region. Just the fact somebody is pampering the little one will help make them feel better.

Cooling remedy

When your child complains of feeling hot and a temperature is looming, this cooling formula can help bring down the heat.

> 1 litre room temperature water
> 2 drops Bosisto's Eucalyptus Oil
> 2 drops lavender oil

Swish these around in a bowl. With a face washer soak in the solution and wipe over head, face and neck area. To make a compress, add 10 drops of eucalyptus oil and 10 drops lavender oil to one litre of warm water. Soak washer and wring out excess water. Compress.

A sheet can be soaked in the compress solution and wrung out. Wrap the little one in it, but be sure it is not too cold; have slightly warm room temperature.

To deter head lice

Funny how we associate lice with dirty hair. Not true! Lice are not fussy about whose head they infect. When you know these six-legged insects are around, it's time to be preventative.

Add a few drops of eucalyptus oil, rosemary and lemon oil to your shampoo and final rinse solution. Brush hair daily or use a fine toothed comb. Nits do not make the head itchy until they have hatched.

Now I'm a teenager

Now the fun begins! My skin looks awful, I hate school – the list becomes endless. A facial scrub can do wonders.

> 10 gms finely ground almonds
> 1/2 teaspoon cinnamon
> 1 raw white of egg
> 6 drops Bosisto's Eucalyptus Oil

Whisk all ingredients together. On a face or back already wet, place mixture into palm of the hand and apply to face. Wash off with a non-perfumed soap. Add a couple of drops of eucalyptus oil to some water and splash face. This can be repeated using fresh mixture a couple of times weekly.

Classroom stress

A blend of some essential oils can help the everyday stresses of classrooms.

> 30 mL sweet almond Oil
> 20 drops Bosisto's Eucalyptus Oil
> 10 drops lemon oil
> 10 drops bergamot oil
> 10 drops lavender oil

Blend together and use as a massage oil over the body, before setting off for school.

Use again at the end of the day.

Around the Home

Purifying

If you are selling your home, having visitors or just love the smell of a clean home, the following will give you an added bonus. Our sense of smell is very powerful and most of us are not aware of how often we utilise this amazing sense. I'm sure that if you are buying a home, walk into one that looks great, but has this awful smell of mould, mildew and other people smells, it can be one big turn-off. Purifying the home with eucalyptus oil will become an everyday event, once you see and gain the benefits of it.

(I use it for absolutely everything. It is my most important cleaning solution. – Cherie).

Famous wool wash recipe

To keep woollens soft and fluffy you will find the following tried and tested recipe to be excellent – try it, you will be convinced.

Pure Soap Flakes	(300˙g)	1/2 packet
Methylated Spirits	(200mL)	1 cup
Bosisto's Eucalyptus Oil	(50mL)	1 small bottle

Mix methylated spirits with soap flakes. Add eucalyptus oil and stir. Store in a wide-necked, screw-capped jar (large coffee jar)

Use one tablespoon mixture per garment. Dissolve in small-quantity hot water and then pour into lukewarm wash water.

Hand or machine wash on wool cycle.

No need to rinse unless white garments are to be stored for a long period (rinsing reduces the risk of yellowing)

Squeeze and roll in towel to remove excess water.

Keep garments in shape while drying out of direct sunlight.

Consumer comments

"I enjoy making our own wool wash mix – prefer to do that than purchase the ready mixed available at the supermarket. My daughter and I both have wool carpet and we use the wool wash to help keep it clean. I have also used it on synthetic carpet with good results. We wash all our cushions and pillows and my dining chairs have gold

velvet cushions – these are successfully washed. My daughter has brown velvet chairs – she uses it to maintain its good looks. I think what I want to say is it's a 'dam' good product."

J.M. WA

"Eucalyptus was always used in my mother's home as it has been in my own. I think the recipe for washing woollens fabulous, occasionally use it in the bathrooms here as I like its refreshing smell. May I add that I find the same combination splendid for tired rheumaticky feet and also for removing hard skin on the soles of my heels. It is very successful for shampooing mats also."

M.S. SA

"I have been hand-spinning wool for some years now and have had some problems in washing the wool clean without felting it. I tried your wool wash recipe and have found that the results have been excellent."

L.C. SA

"I use a great amount of Bosisto's Oil of Eucalyptus for making up mixtures of wool mix. I have sheep and spin the fleece and use this mixture for washing the wool as a final step in cleaning it. I also have great use of it in the household."

G.O. Vic

"Sometimes spinning wheels are left with me for cleaning and maintenance and I have been asked what I use to clean the metal orifice where the greasy wool fleece is fed through when spinning yarn. I dip a cotton bud into Bosisto's Eucalyptus Oil – its amazing how much grime and build up it removes."

J.L. WA

"I used some eucalyptus oil in a bowl of Softly recently to remove some bad stains on a jumper – after dry-cleaning fluid had failed – and it worked perfectly."

A.P. SA

Bathroom

To clean the tiles in the bathroom and shower area the
following recipe is ideal.

> Pure soap flakes around cup to 1 bucket hot
> water.
> 1/2 cup methylated spirits
> 25 mL Bosisto's Eucalyptus Oil

Swish these through the water, use a brush to remove
excess build-up. Repeat process if necessary. Rinse off
with warm water.

The washing woollens recipe can also be used.

Consumer comment

*"My husband does not like the artificial
aromas of any (and all) air fresheners for
toilet and bathroom. In despair I noticed
your Eucalyptus Spray on the shop shelf and
decided to try it! Eureka!! Since then I have
also cleaned spots from the camper,
dry-cleaned marks from suits and trousers –
as well as used it to relieve muscle pain at
times."*

M.S. NSW

Mould and mildew

Bathroom   Use hot soapy water and add a capful of eucalyptus oil. Use the spray in between washing.

Bedroom   You can generally smell the mildew in the cupboards. Use hot soapy water where possible and then spray liberally the area with eucalyptus spray.

Shoes   Clean shoes with a damp cloth and eucalyptus oil. In an old stocking, place some pot-pourri and a teaspoonful of eucalyptus oil. Stuff it into shoes that are not worn regularly. This is also ideal for smelly shoes and after sport, when they get a little offensive.

Clothes   Wash with woollen wash mix or add two capfuls to the wash.

Bench tops

Spray Bosisto's Eucalyptus on benches and tabletops. For a stronger solution use some detergent, hot water and a teaspoon of eucalyptus oil.

Bedroom

One of the most lived-in places in the home deserves to be clean and smell good.

(I wipe over with a damp cloth and eucalyptus oil all the dust-collecting areas – from the bed head to the cupboard. – Cherie).

Use the eucalyptus spray on the mattress each time you change the sheets. Spray the pillows and the carpet. Not only does it purify the room but it also acts as an insect deterrent.

Consumer comment

> *"I find Bosisto's Eucalyptus Spray a great product for all the reasons you have on the can plus mildewed wardrobes, smokey rooms, smelly running shoes."*
>
> *D.C. NSW*

Anti-moth treatment

Blend together one teaspoon eucalyptus oil, one teaspoon lavender oil, one teaspoon lemon oil; shake well. Place a few drops on to padded coat hangers;

sprinkle on drawer liners. When cleaning cupboards, wipe over with damp cloth and a few drops of mixture.

Silverfish

Wipe shelves with eucalyptus oil.

Carpet freshener

Consumer comment

> *"I have been making a simple carpet freshener by mixing bi-carb soda with eucalyptus oil."*

S.D. Vic

> *"I mixed your eucalyptus oil – about 25mL to 500g bi-carb soda and sprinkled on carpet and left one hour and it helped my flea problem in the carpets and smelt nice too."*

W.N. Qld

Vacuum cleaner

Consumer comment

> "Two other things I use the oil for is : 1 – a
> few drops on the filter of my vacuum cleaner
> and the same on my clothes dryer. The
> warm air coming out sends a lovely
> eucalyptus aroma through the house. 2 –
> being a non-smoker I hate dirty ashtrays,
> especially in my car. When I clean them out,
> I leave a cotton ball with a few drops of oil
> inside. When opened, it puts people off from
> using them and makes the car smell clean".

S.A. Vic

Crew quarters

Consumer comment

> "We use Bosisto's Eucalyptus Spray to
> disinfect and deodorise fishing trawlers
> accommodation".

N.M. Qld

Fragrant candles and aromatisers

To keep the home smelling fresh and clean for hours on end, an aromatiser can be the answer. Pharmacies sell a Euky Bear Vaporiser. This is ideal for colds and stuffy noses, little ones with croup and bronchial conditions. Not only does it help those who are ill, the home will also have a very pleasant aroma permeating and this will help to prevent everyone else becoming ill.

Electric Burners	Add around 10 drops of eucalyptus oil.
Candles	Add 1-2 drops before lighting candle. (Keep out of reach of children)

Air conditioners can be a health hazard. Be sure to clean the filter regularly, wash in soapy water, then rinse with clean water and one teaspoonful of eucalyptus oil. For the office and workplace these can be a great prevention against disease.

Evaporitve water coolers – add some eucalyptus oil to the water.

A Gardeners Delight

Garden Spray Recipe

Eucalyptus Garden Spray has become very popular with home gardeners because it is organic and safe to use. You can mix your own spray by using the easy-to-make formula set out below:

Canola Oil	20mL
Bosisto's Eucalyptus Oil	5mL
Dishwashing detergent (any good brand)	2mL
Water	1 litre

Consumers have reported it is very good on aphids, white flies and mites. Apply spray when they first appear. Apply two sprays three to five days apart. Repeat applications if there is re-infestation. Use up to double the concentration if the numbers are high. Thoroughly spray the foliage to run off. Use on roses, azaleas, tomatoes, cucumbers, strawberries etc.

Do not store made up spray. Wash sprayer after use.

Snail repellent

To keep snails and slugs out of the garden, fill a saucer or lid with water and add 10 drops of eucalyptus oil. Place a few of these around the garden. Snails hate rough surfaces. Spread some chip bark around the border of the garden.

Insect repellent

Pieces of string can be soaked in eucalyptus oil then wound around areas where seedlings or plants are being attacked. Repeat every couple of days.

Bosisto's Eucalyptus Oil is a good for keeping mosquitos away. As eucalyptus oil burns like kerosene, try the oil alone or mixed with kerosene in flares and lanterns. These can be placed beside the pond or around the garden. Ideal when outdoors for a barbecue. After using your barbecue, clean the plate with hot soapy water, eucalyptus oil (around one teaspoonful) and a scourer or steel wool. Rinse off thoroughly.

Garden Ponds

As lovely as they look, they can be a great breeding ground for mosquito's and other creepy crawlies. Buy an artificial flower or water lily, place a few drops of eucalyptus oil on to it and let it float in the pond.

Insect repelling body oil

Canola oil contains one of natures best-kept secrets, it contains a natural chemical that repels insects.

Blend into 100mL canola oil, 30 drops eucalyptus oil, 10 drops basil oil, 10 drops citronella oil. Apply a little to the palm of the hand, rub and warm, smooth over exposed areas. Re-apply every two to three hours. This can also be applied to a brush or comb and used on your cat or dog. Only use a couple of drops on the brush or comb.

Consumer comment

> "For many years I have used the following personal insect repellent:
>
> 1 part eucalyptus oil
> 1 part methylated spirits
> 1 part cider vinegar

*I place directly into a bottle with a smallish
opening. Shake well before applying to skin.
Good against mosquitoes and flies."*

B.S. Qld

Bee stings

Remove the sting and dab eucalyptus oil on to the
area.

Consumer comment

*"I would like to tell you that I have been
using Eucalyptus Oil for nearly 60 years and
my mother used it before me. One use we
used it for was bee stings when we were
stung and we had over 1000 hives so we had
a few stings."*

L.N. Vic

Sunburn

Make up a solution of green tea. Leave it go cold and
place around 100ml into a spritzer. Add one
teaspoonful of eucalyptus oil, shake well. Spray on to
affected areas.

Cuts and scratches

A gentle prick from a rose thorn can become a major infection. Remove thorn and soak in warm water and eucalyptus oil. Repeat process every couple of hours. Cuts and scratches from branches and twigs can be washed with warm water and eucalyptus oil, around 5 mL per two litres of water.

Grass stains

Soak the stain in eucalyptus oil for at least one hour before washing.

Repotting

When repotting it is essential to clean bacteria from pots before the new plant is put in. With hot soapy water and a teaspoonful of eucalyptus oil, wash the pot out thoroughly. Rinse well.

Outside Maintenance

Garden tools

Clean garden tools in hot water and eucalyptus oil. This helps to eliminate bacteria that can create cross-contamination in the soils.

Garbage bins

Wash regularly with hot soapy water and eucalyptus oil. Use the spray in between washing.

Grease and stains

Our cars and equipment can leave quite a mess in the garage or carport. This can build up to dangerous proportions. With hot soapy water, 10ml of eucalyptus oil and a scrubbing brush, clean the area.

Paint stains

When painting window frames etc, remove any drops that may have landed where you don't need them, with a little eucalyptus oil on a damp cloth.

Windows

To clean very dirty windows, spray eucalyptus oil over them, wipe over with damp newspaper. This is also fantastic for the mirrors, particularly when they fog up. Wash mirror with methylated spirits or vinegar and water, wipe over with eucalyptus on damp newspaper. This will minimise fogging.

Penetrating oil

Consumer comment

> *"We find the eucalyptus oil also very good for loosening rust on nuts."*

> *D.K. Qld*

Car radiators

Consumers who have used eucalyptus oil in radiators say it is quite good for controlling rust. When radiators are old and showing signs of rust, add two tablespoons (25mL-30mL) eucalyptus oil and run the engine until the water is rusty. Flush out and repeat the process until the water is clear. (Two flushings should be sufficient). Fill the radiator with clean water, add two tablespoons eucalyptus oil. If the water shows rust again in six months or so, repeat the process.

(We advise that eucalyptus oil is a strong solvent and may soften rubber if left in contact with it for long periods. As Felton, Grimwade & Bickford has not performed tests on radiators, we would suggest you confine experiments to older vehicles).

Possums in roof

Some consumers note that a rag soaked in eucalyptus oil and left in the roof keeps possums away. Re-soak rag from time to time.

Leeches

A consumer suggested Bosisto's Eucalyptus Oil sprayed inside leggings or on clothing or skin will keep leeches at bay. There is a certain irony about this as Felton Grimwade traded in leeches in the 1870's and 1880's. Aborigines caught the leeches by wading into the swamps around Echuca. They were sent to the company's specially built aquarium in Melbourne and then taken by passenger ship to England, France and America. There were complaints from passengers about leeches escaping and attaching themselves to ladies in their cabins. It is a pity the ladies were unaware of the use of Bosisto's Eucalyptus Oil.

Caring for Pets

Our domestic friends become part of the family. They also suffer with many complaints that we do, except they can't tell us. We generally can tell if our dog has a cough or a cold, is scratching excessively, or that something is not quite right.

Firstly, their environment needs to be kept clean and free from creepy crawlies. Animals have a keen sense of smell, so always use the minimum amount of essential oils.

Fleas and parasites

Into around two cups of warm water place four drops eucalyptus oil and two drops cedarwood. Dip brush into water and brush coat, repeating this with clean applications, several times. Rinse well with warm water. This helps to remove the eggs as well as fleas and parasites. Wash all bedding in eucalyptus oil, soap flakes and warm water.

A flea collar can also help. Apply a few drops of eucalyptus oil and two drops of citronella oil, blend this in a teaspoon of vegetable oil and rub well on collar. Repeat this every few days.

Arthritis

If your dog is suffering from arthritis, make up a blend to help the joints. It will help if you can gently massage this into the affected area.

> 50 ml olive oil
> 5 drops eucalyptus oil

Blend these together, massage well into area. By the time the dog may start to lick this oil, the essential oil will have penetrated. This is quite safe.

Cats can be treated the same as for dogs, but always remember not to overdose your pet with any essential oils.

Shampoo

Two to three drops of eucalyptus oil and one drop of lavender oil can be added to your pet's shampoo and conditioner.

Pet quarters

Spray area around sleeping quarters with eucalyptus spray; allow for the oil to disperse before allowing your pet back. Wash all eating utensils with detergent and eucalyptus oil. Soak them in this solution if they have been out in the sun all day.

Consumer comments

> *We have been using Bosisto's Eucalyptus Oil in the surgery as a general disinfectant/deodoriser for the past five years."*
>
> Dr R. Vet WA

> *"I began raising squirrel Glider Possums from extreme infancy and thanks to my many years of hard work, was successful. I use pure eucalyptus oil (Bosisto's) and have used same from the onset as a disinfectant for their quarters."*
>
> J.P. Qld.

*"Bosisto's Eucalyptus Oil, we use for the
hygienic cleaning and natural smell of pens,
boxes and bedding for the animals in our
care. We have found Bosisto's Eucalyptus Oil
of great benefit for the safety and well-being
of the animals."*

Wildlife Welfare Agency – Qld.

*"Bosisto's 'Parrot' Brand Eucalyptus Spray is
an excellent product. It is particularly useful
in wafting away dog odours from my car."*

L.T. Qld

Cuts and scratches

Add six drops of eucalyptus oil to warm water and
bathe. Blend two drops of eucalyptus oil into some
aloe vera gel and apply to area. Bandage, if possible,
until it begins to heal.

Bird cages

Wash trays and utensils with hot, soapy water and
around one teaspoonful eucalyptus oil. Rinse off well.

Flies

Soak pieces of ribbon in eucalyptus oil and tie onto bird cage, and areas where flies are lurking.

Coughs and colds

A blend to massage on to the chest of your pet will certainly help when they are feeling yuk! Blend two to five drops of eucalyptus oil into 50mL grapeseed oil. If you have a very small pet, use a lesser amount.

Rabbits and hamsters

Their homes must be kept clean and dry. Use eucalyptus oil and detergent with hot water, to wash the cages. This helps to prevent infections and keep them healthy.

Horses

Stables attract mice, so these areas must be kept very clean. Make up a mixture in a bucket with two capfuls of eucalyptus oil, a good dash of detergent and fill with hot water. If mice are present, add 10 drops of peppermint oil.

Flies also like to hang around stables. Place three drops of eucalyptus oil and three drops of citronella oil on to a brush and brush the horse's coat. This will help to deter the flies.

Compresses are ideal for horses. It is so important to quickly heal injuries to the legs, and this helps to speed up the healing process from strains, bruises and fractures.

> 100mL olive oil
> 10 drops Bosisto's Eucalyptus Oil
> 10 drops ginger oil.

Blend this together and compress on to leg. Place a cabbage leaf over oil blend and then bandage. Continue compressing after healing to strengthen the ligaments and prevent calcification.

Consumer comment

> *"Years ago my husband, who lived on a sheep station, also had horses. One horse that had strangles, he treated with eucalyptus in bran in a nose bag and after a time the horse improved. He is sure it was through using the eucalyptus".*

Travel Tips

(Whenever I travel I take my eucalyptus oil with me. For ear pressure, a few drops on a hanky and inhaled will help greatly. Often when I reach my destination, the room may have an unpleasant or stale odour. Out with the eucalyptus spray or oil and the room feels – and is – much more pleasant. – Cherie).

Feet can be a problem, particularly if they have become swollen during flight. Use a wet face cloth with a liberal amount of eucalyptus oil on it and place over the feet. When you reach your destination, have a footbath with eucalyptus oil in it. Your feet will feel refreshed and the swelling subsides much more quickly.

Jetlag can spoil a journey. Once you have reached your destination, have an aromatic bath with eucalyptus oil, drink some lemon or grapefruit juice, and you will be much more refreshed.

Before you set off on a journey, wet a handkerchief and sprinkle with eucalyptus oil. Place in an airtight plastic bag. When feeling tired or congested, open the bag and inhale.

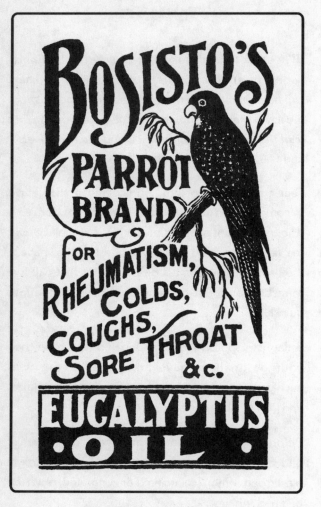

A Bosisto label, around 1916.

Precautions and Safety

Paracelsus (1493-1541), the Swiss physician whose radical ideas influenced the development of medicine, wrote in about 1530 *"all things are poisons. It is only the dose which make a thing poison"*. Even water and salt which are normally harmless may cause illness or death if taken in excess.

Eucalyptus oil is very concentrated. It is the essence of the tree. It needs to be used sparingly and with care.

Although eucalyptus oil is toxic if ingested in excessive quantities, Australia is the only country in the world to legislate that products containing 25 per cent or more eucalyptus oil must be labelled poison and packed in a poison container. The container must be sealed with a child-resistant closure.

Products containing less than 25% eucalyptus oil can be sold without having to be labelled poison, without having to be packed in poison containers and without being sealed with a child-resistant closure. Their use is not restricted in any way.

Manufacturers often incorporate eucalyptus oil into cough lozenges, cough syrups, toothpastes, mouth washes and as a flavour ingredient in foods.

Home-made oral preparations containing pure eucalyptus oil are not recommended unless the measurement of the amount of eucalyptus oil used is very accurate. The highly respected and authoritative German Commission E monograph on eucalyptus oil under 'Dosage' states, for internal use, a daily dose of 0.3 to 0.6g.

It is perfectly safe to take eucalyptus orally provided the dosage is kept within this use range. It is not advisable to take eucalyptus oil over a long period (a year or more) as it may cause liver damage.

The acute oral toxicity LD50 of eucalyptus oil for rats is 2.48g/kg body weight. Evidence indicates the LD50 for humans is probably about the same. There have been no reported deaths due to the ingestion of eucalyptus oil in the past 50 years.

Where accidental poisoning has occurred there have been no reports of long-term side effects. Other household products such as paracetamol, oil of wintergreen, methyl salicylate, kerosene and petrol have proved to be much more dangerous.

The acute dermal toxicity of eucalyptus oil exceeds 5g/kg body weight. A patch test using full-strength eucalyptus oil for 24 hours produced no reaction in 20 subjects. Ten per cent of eucalyptus oil in petrolatum produced no irritation in a 48-hour closed patch test in 25 human subjects. This means most people will not have any adverse reaction from eucalyptus oil when applied to the skin.

Very occasionally hypersensitivity has been reported in susceptible individuals. Anyone who is hypersensitive should cease using the product immediately. There have been no reports of phototoxicity (sensitivity to light).

Flammability

Eucalyptus oil is about as flammable as kerosene so keep it away from heat, spark and flame.

Caution

As eucalyptus oil is very concentrated, avoid contact with eyes, mucous membranes, lips, tongue, polished furniture, some plastic surfaces and some materials such as denim, silk and non-colourfast materials. Patch test before using.

Historical Bottles

Alfred Felton and Frederick Grimwade established the Melbourne Bottle Works in 1872 to supply bottles to their expanding wholesale drug business and to meet the growing needs of the community. Importing glass bottles was proving to be difficult, uncertain, expensive and inconvenient, so local manufacture seemed to be a better solution.

While the first few years proved difficult, the company went from a small-bottle works to Australia's fourth largest public company when it was known as Australian Glass Manufacturers (AGM) It became Australian Consolidated Industries (ACI) in 1939.

Many of the bottles produced during the early years survive today. One of the earliest bottles produced was for Bosisto's Eucalyptus Oil.

People often dig bottles up in their gardens. Antique bottle enthusiasts are more than likely to have one or more in their collections.

The markings on the bottles indicate when they were manufactured. Some of the markings and dates are as follows:

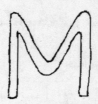

Melbourne Glass Bottle Works

1872 – 1916

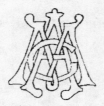

AGM Company

1916 - 1932

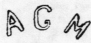

OR

1923 – 1930

1930 – today

Letters on bottles indicating year of manufacture

(mostly for beers and soft drinks)

E	1928	⊓	1941	4	1954	7	1967
F	1929	Ǝ	1942	5	1955	8	1968
G	1930	Ⅎ	1943	6	1956	9	1969
H	1931	⅁	1944	7	1957	0	1970
J	1932	⊥	1945	8	1958	1	1971
K	1933	6	1946	9	1959	2	1972
L	1934	7	1947	0	1960	3	1973
M	1935	8	1948	1	1961	4	1974
N	1936	9	1949	2	1962	5	1975
D	1937	0	1950	3	1963	6	1976
A	1938	1	1951	4	1964	7	1977
Ꞵ	1939	2	1952	5	1965	8	1978
Ɔ	1940	3	1953	6	1966	9	1979
						0	1980

Examples

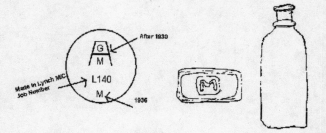

Index

Eucalyptus Oil Uses, Hints and Recipes

For more information contact:

Felton Grimwade & Bickford Pty Ltd
61 Clarinda Road
Oakleigh South
Victoria 3167 Australia
Phone: (03) 9562 7711
Fax: (03) 9562 7291
Email: mail@fgb.com.au
Website: www.fgb.com.au